Herbal Remedies for Cancer

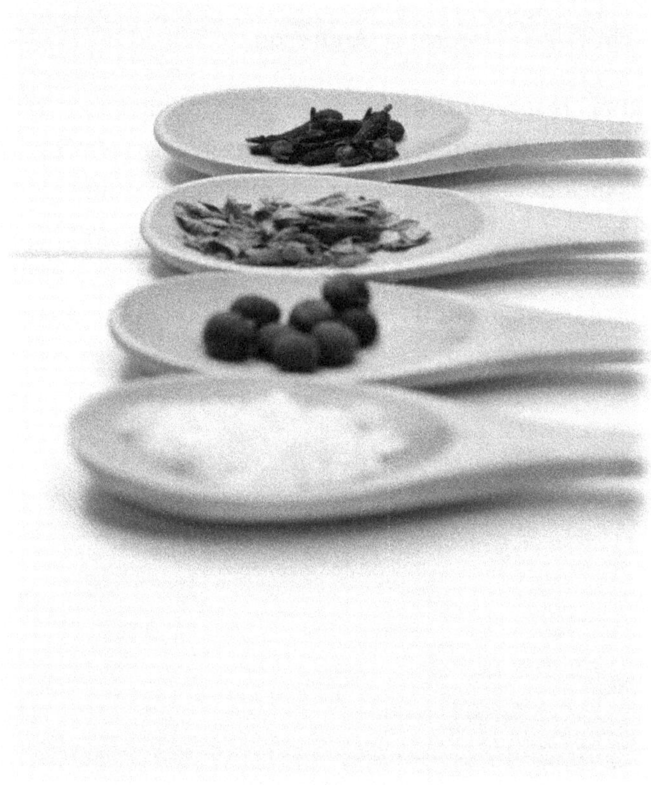

Hector A Anderson

Table of Contents

Introduction

A cancer diagnosis is an emotional and life-changing experience that necessitates fortitude, education, and a holistic approach to well-being. "Herbal Remedies for Cancer" is more than a handbook; it's a companion, a source of information, and a beacon of hope for people traversing the difficult terrain of cancer and its therapies.

What exactly is cancer?

Cancer, at its heart, is a complicated and deadly foe—a group of illnesses characterized by the uncontrolled development and spread of aberrant cells. This book begins by demystifying cancer, explaining its numerous kinds, phases of progression, and ramifications for individuals and their loved ones. With this knowledge, you'll be able to make more educated decisions about your recovery path.

The Emotional Repercussions

Cancer has a tremendous emotional impact that cannot be exaggerated, in addition to its physical symptoms. Fear, uncertainty, and stress accompany you on this trip, hurting your mental health and general quality of life. Recognizing and dealing with the emotional toll is critical. This book recognizes the necessity of managing not just the medical elements of cancer, but also the complex emotional landscape that comes with the diagnosis.

The emotional rollercoaster that follows, from the first shock of diagnosis to the continuous challenges of therapy, needs a comprehensive approach to well-being. Understanding the emotional elements of cancer is more than simply a prelude to the guide's content; it is a critical component of the advice and assistance provided inside these pages.

The Function of Complementary Therapies

The relevance of complementary medicines in cancer therapy cannot be emphasized. While traditional treatments such as surgery, chemotherapy, and radiation target cancer cells directly, alternative therapies such as herbal medicines take a more holistic approach. They go beyond physical symptoms to address the individual as a whole—mind, body, and soul.

Herbal treatments, in particular, have a long history of usage and are recognized for their anti-inflammatory, antioxidant, and immune-boosting effects. However, it is critical to approach these therapies with knowledge. This guidance highlights that herbal therapies are designed to supplement and enhance the entire care plan rather than to replace conventional medical advice and treatments.

Taking the Herbal Odyssey

As we begin this journey together, it is critical to understand that this book is not a one-size-fits-all answer. Each person's cancer experience is unique, and measures to controlling the disease should be adapted accordingly. "Herbal Remedies for Cancer" aims to educate you on the benefits of adopting herbal medicines with conventional therapy.

Our objective is to provide assistance by providing advise on herbal therapies, dietary considerations, lifestyle changes, and the delicate balance necessary when combining these factors with the recommendations of your healthcare team. We urge you to think of this book as a tool in your toolbox—an educational companion aimed to improve your comprehension, enable interactions with healthcare providers, and help you make well-informed decisions on your route to healing.

In the following chapters, we will look at specific herbs with anti-cancer properties, delve into the art of making herbal infusions, discuss dietary guidelines, look at lifestyle changes, and provide real-life case studies of people who have found success incorporating herbal remedies into their cancer care journey.

Allow us to traverse the difficulties of cancer together, equipped with information, compassion, and the collective power that comes from a community of people dedicated to holistic well-being. The path may be difficult, but there is hope for a happier, healthier future with educated decisions and a thorough strategy.

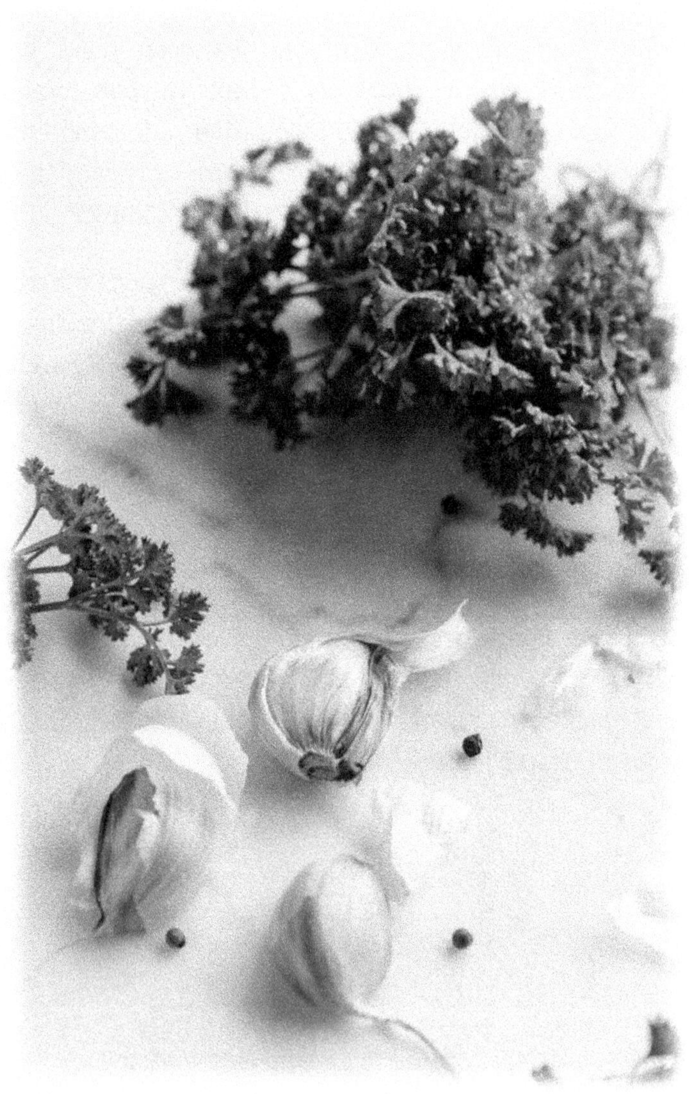

Chapter 1

Decoding Cancer's Complexity: Causes, Types, and Stages

Cancer, a complicated labyrinth of biological aberrations, tests our comprehension and fortitude. To understand this multidimensional foe, we must travel through its roots, its forms, and the developing stages that determine its evolution.

Cancer's Mysterious Causes

The formation of cancer frequently includes a symphony of elements, changing healthy cells into rebels that refuse to obey the body's regulatory processes. Untangling the mystery of causes takes us into the delicate dance of heredity and environment.

Genetic Predisposition: In certain cases, the cellular script contains an error. Certain forms of cancer can be predisposed to by genetic mutations acquired from one's parents. However, it is important to emphasize that not everyone with a genetic susceptibility develops cancer, and environmental factors play a significant impact.

Environmental Factors: Our surrounds are a jumble of possible triggers. Carcinogens, radiation, and some diseases can all cause cellular revolt. Tobacco use, poor eating habits, and sedentary living are all protagonists in this story, and they may all contribute to cellular discord.

Cancer Types

Cancer is not a single illness, but rather a group of diseases, each with its own set of traits, behaviors, and difficulties. The variety of cancer kinds is both encouraging and intimidating.

Breast Cancer: Breast cancer is the most frequent cancer in women worldwide, and it can appear in a variety of ways, underlining the need of early identification and personalized treatment options.

Lung Cancer: A major worldwide health concern, lung cancer is mostly associated with tobacco use. Nonsmokers, on the other hand, might be vulnerable, reflecting the complexities of its origins.

Prostate Cancer: Prostate cancer, which affects the male reproductive system, can range from slow-growing to aggressive, demanding individualized treatment options.

Cancer of the Colon: Colorectal cancer, which arises from the colon or rectum, emphasizes the necessity of screening and lifestyle changes.

Each variety of cancer has its own set of features, necessitating tailored methods to diagnosis, treatment, and survivor care.

Journey Through Cancer Stages

Understanding cancer's course entails navigating through various phases, which are similar to chapters in a book, with each stage revealing new obstacles and complications.

Stage I: The first act, in which cancer is localized and frequently restricted to the site of genesis. Treatment at this point usually has a positive effect.

Stage II: The narrative thickens as cancer spreads beyond its original site, posing new hurdles for successful treatment.

Stage III: The intrusion of neighboring tissues and lymph nodes heightens the drama. Strategic therapies are required to halt its progression.

Stage IV: The last stage of metastasis, in which cancer has spread to distant organs. As finding a cure becomes increasingly difficult, management concentrates on quality of life.

The origins, kinds, and stages of cancer weave a complicated story that necessitates an informed and adaptable response. As we explore deeper into the complexities of this foe, it becomes evident that the route to understanding cancer is not linear—it is a dynamic journey requiring constant investigation and adaptation.

Demystifying Conventional Treatments

In the continuous war against this complicated opponent, conventional cancer therapies constitute a powerful armament. As we continue on the road of demystifying these treatments, it is critical to shed light on their underlying principles, potential adverse effects, and the critical role they play in the search of healing.

1. Surgery: Precision in Intervention

Surgery is one of the oldest and most direct ways of cancer treatment. Consider it a sculptor's chisel, methodically cutting out the cancer. Whether removing a tumor, lymph nodes, or an entire organ, surgery strives for accuracy, excising malignant tissues while leaving healthy ones alone. Technological advancements, such as less invasive treatments, improve both efficacy and recuperation durations.

2. Chemotherapy for Rapid Growth

Chemotherapy, which is sometimes seen as the frontline infantry in cancer treatment, entails using strong medications to inhibit the fast division of cancer cells. Consider it a methodical attack on the battlefield, with cells targeted wherever they may be in the body. While chemotherapy is extremely successful, it is also renowned for causing collateral damage to healthy cells, resulting in side effects like as hair loss, nausea, and tiredness. Individualizing treatment regimens aids in striking a fine balance between effectiveness and limiting side effects.

3. Radiation Therapy: Precision from Afar

Radiation treatment uses high doses of radiation to selectively target and destroy cancer cells. Consider it as a sniper shooting for the enemy's heart. Precision is improved by technological improvements like as intensity-modulated radiation treatment (IMRT) and proton therapy, which minimizes harm to adjacent healthy tissues. Fatigue and localized skin responses are common side effects that are usually transitory.

4. Immunotherapy: Mobilizing the Body's Defenses

Immunotherapy, which uses the body's immune system to detect and attack cancer cells, marks a paradigm change in cancer treatment. Consider it like training the body's own warriors to identify and eliminate intruders. This method has demonstrated great effectiveness, particularly in some tumors, with fewer side effects than usual therapies.

5. Hormone Therapy: Restricting Cancer's Fuel

Hormone treatment tries to deny cancer cells of the hormones they require to proliferate in hormone-driven malignancies such as breast and prostate cancer. Consider it like shutting off a fire's fuel source. Hormone treatment, while typically well-tolerated, might cause hot flashes, lethargy, and libido problems.

6. Targeted Therapy: Precision Strikes

Targeted treatment is analogous to launching smart missiles at specific weaknesses within cancer cells. These treatments strive for maximum impact with little collateral damage to healthy tissues by focusing on particular properties of cancer cells. The most common adverse effects differ according on the targeted treatment utilized.

Conventional cancer therapies, which are sometimes viewed as strong opponents in their own right, are effective weapons in the fight for recovery. While they can result in spectacular accomplishments, it is critical to note that they may also provide problems along the road. The key is to have a thorough awareness of each treatment method, to communicate openly with healthcare personnel, and to recognize that the landscape of cancer care is changing.

As we deconstruct these standard therapies, it becomes clear that they are not stand-alone answers, but rather components of a wider, more comprehensive approach to cancer care. In the following sections, we'll look at the possible synergy between conventional therapies and herbal cures, as well as dietary concerns and lifestyle changes. Let us unravel the complexity together, equipped with information and a comprehensive viewpoint on the path to healing.

Managing Treatment Side Effects

The route to cancer therapy is fraught with difficulties, not the least of which are the side effects that frequently accompany the vigorous treatments aimed at battling the disease. Understanding and controlling these side effects are critical components of holistic cancer treatment.

1. Embracing the Fundamentals: Hydration and self-care

Fatigue: A frequent companion on this road, tiredness may be crippling. Rest first, listen to your body, and divide chores into small bits. Gentle activity, such as walking, can also help with weariness.

Hydration: Many negative effects can be exacerbated by dehydration. Stay hydrated, especially if nausea or vomiting are a problem. Drinking water throughout the day and eating hydrated meals may make a big impact.

2. Addressing Gastrointestinal Issues

Nausea and Vomiting: Anti-nausea drugs recommended by your healthcare team can successfully treat these adverse effects. Smaller, more frequent meals, as well as avoiding strong scents, can also assist.

Diarrhea and Constipation: Bowel changes are prevalent. Constipation can be helped with a high-fiber diet, whereas diarrhea can be helped with anti-diarrheal drugs and dietary changes.

3. Tackling Hair Loss

The possibility of hair loss may be emotionally taxing for many people. Consider wearing wigs, scarves, or other head coverings that make you feel comfortable and confident. Remember that hair frequently regrows following treatment.

4. Coping with Changes in Appetite and Taste

Chemotherapy and other treatments might cause changes in your taste and appetite. Experimenting with different cuisines, flavors, and textures may help you learn what foods, spices, and textures appeal to your taste buds. A healthy diet is essential for general well-being.

5. Handling Skin Changes

Skin changes can be caused by radiation treatment and certain drugs. Use mild, fragrance-free products on your skin and keep it hydrated. Avoid direct sun exposure and notify your healthcare provider of any changes that are worrying.

6. Navigating Emotional and Cognitive Changes

Cancer therapies can have an effect on emotions and cognitive function. Seek help from mental health specialists, participate in support groups, and employ stress-reduction practices such as meditation and mindfulness.

Communication is Key:

Communication with your healthcare staff should be open and honest. They can offer customized methods and, if necessary, modify your treatment plan to reduce adverse effects. Never be afraid to express your concerns or seek advice.

Integrating Complementary Therapies:

Under the supervision of your healthcare team, investigate alternative therapies such as herbal medicines and acupuncture. Some people find that these measures help them manage side effects and improve their general well-being.

Building a Support Network:

Surround yourself with a solid support network—friends, family, and support groups may offer emotional as well as practical support. When you need them, don't be afraid to call on them.

Treatment side effects management is a continuous and customized procedure. Every person's path is unique, and solutions that work for one person may not work for another. The goal is to have open lines of communication with your healthcare team, practice self-care, and seek support from people around you. Remember that managing side effects is an important element of the holistic approach to recovery as you traverse the landscape of cancer treatment.

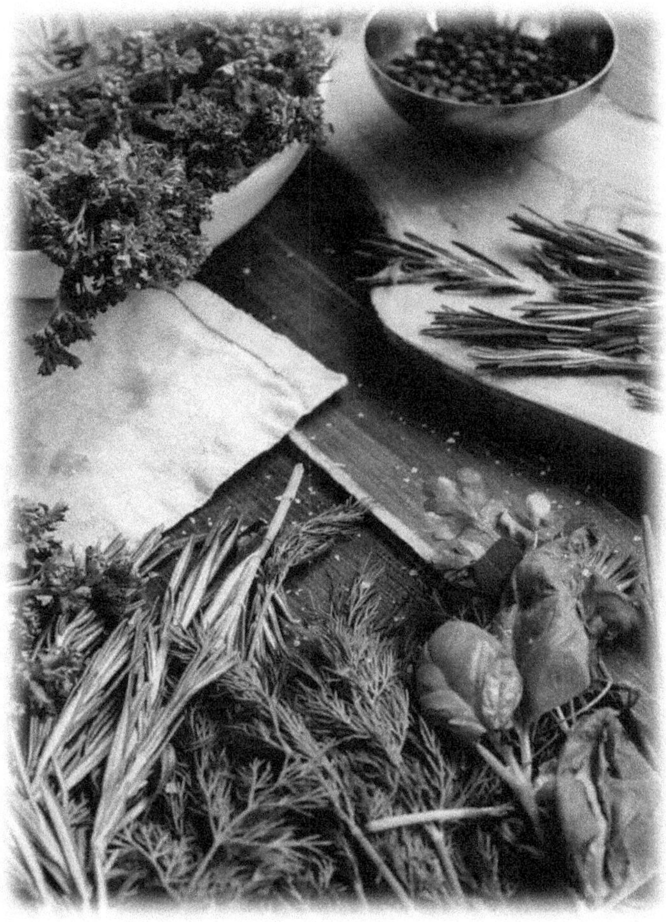

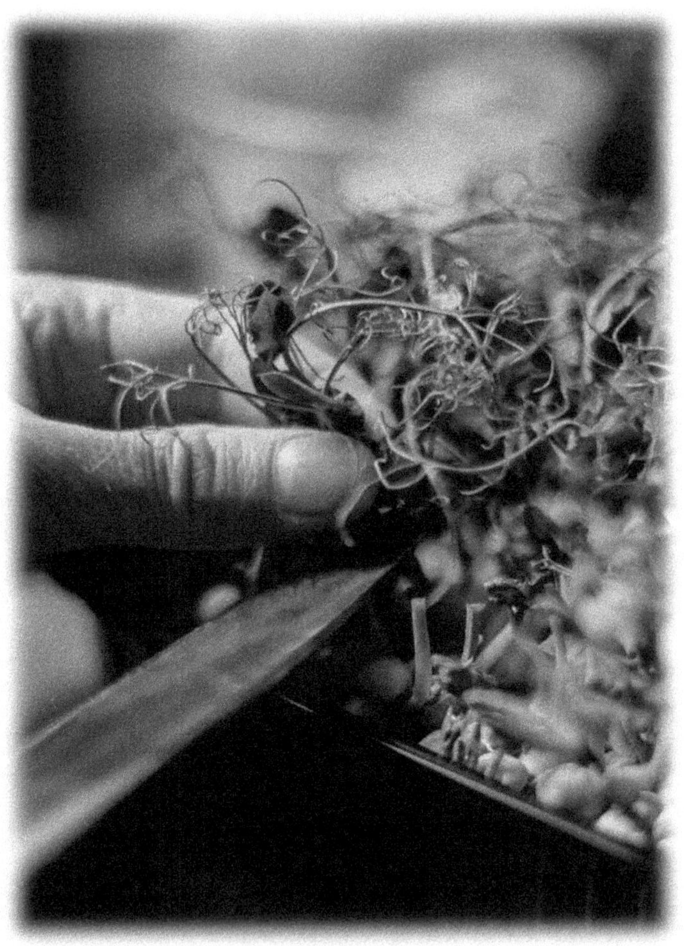

Chapter 2

Herbal Remedies' Role in Cancer Treatment

As we traverse the complex terrain of cancer treatment, the attention is increasingly shifting to the age-old knowledge of herbal medicines. Herbal medicine's function in cancer therapy goes beyond simple tradition, into a domain where nature's offers play an important role in supporting and strengthening conventional medicines.

1. Utilizing Nature's Pharmacy

Herbal medicine, which is steeped in millennia of cultural and medical practices, encapsulates the essence of utilizing plants' therapeutic power. Consider it a trip to nature's pharmacy, where chemicals found in plants have a wide range of medicinal effects. Herbs include a varied array of bioactive substances that have promise in the battle against cancer, ranging from anti-inflammatory and antioxidant properties to immune system regulation.

2. Synergy with Conventional Treatments

The potential synergy with conventional therapies is one of the most important features of incorporating herbal medicines into cancer therapy. Herbal treatment, while not a replacement for surgery, chemotherapy, or radiation, can supplement traditional procedures. Certain herbs, for example, may improve the efficiency of chemotherapy or reduce its negative effects, allowing for a more holistic approach to care.

3. Immune System Aid

The immune system is critical in recognizing and destroying aberrant cells, including cancer cells. Herbal medicines include immunomodulatory effects, which help the body's natural defensive processes. Herbs such as echinacea, astragalus, and medicinal mushrooms are thought to boost immune function, making the environment less favorable for cancer formation and progression.

4. Targeting Inflammation and Oxidative Stress

Chronic inflammation and oxidative stress have been linked to cancer development and progression. Herbal treatments, which are high in anti-inflammatory and antioxidant ingredients, can help with these issues. Turmeric, which contains curcumin, and green tea, which contains polyphenols, are two plants that have shown anti-inflammatory and antioxidant properties in preclinical research.

5. Reducing Treatment negative Effects

Herbs can help manage the negative effects of conventional cancer therapies. For example, ginger may aid with nausea linked with chemotherapy, while peppermint may help with digestive difficulties. When combined with conventional therapy, these natural remedies contribute to a more holistic and patient-centered approach.

6. Individualized Approaches

Herbal therapy emphasizes the uniqueness of each individual's health profile. The holistic viewpoint recognizes that different people respond differently to therapies. Herbal medicines provide for a more tailored approach, taking into account not just the specific cancer type but also the individual's general health, genetics, and unique demands.

7. Caution and Collaboration with Healthcare Professionals

While the potential advantages of herbal treatments in cancer therapy are appealing, they must be approached with caution. Certain plants may have drug interactions or be contraindicated. Collaboration with healthcare experts is critical for the safe use of herbal treatments into a complete treatment plan. Open communication enables educated decisions and coordinated care.

8. Patient Empowerment and Well-Being

Herbal treatments, in addition to their potential physiological effects, empower patients on their cancer journey. Herb usage promotes a sense of proactive engagement in one's health, which contributes to general well-being. This empowerment extends beyond the physical domain to include emotional and mental components of healing.

Herbal medicines' function in cancer treatment is a complex and changing story. Herbal therapy, which is rooted in tradition and increasingly backed by scientific research, provides a holistic viewpoint that matches with the delicate nature of cancer care.

As we continue to investigate this area, the synergy between herbal therapies and conventional treatments appears as a viable path for improving the overall well-being of cancer patients.

The Crucial Importance of Combining Herbs with Conventional Treatments in Cancer Care

The symbiotic interaction between herbal medicines and conventional therapies emerges as a critical component in the complicated tapestry of cancer care, enabling a holistic and integrated approach to recovery. Understanding the significance of merging these two modalities is critical, as it reveals a story in which the whole is genuinely more than the sum of its parts.

1. Increasing Treatment Efficacy

Combining herbal therapies with conventional treatments generates a synergy that can improve cancer care's overall efficacy. While surgery, chemotherapy, radiation, and other conventional therapies directly target cancer cells, herbal medicines can function as supporting agents, potentially improving the efficacy of these treatments. This joint method combines the best of both worlds in order to provide a complete and powerful response to the complexities of cancer.

2. Reducing Treatment Side Effects

Conventional cancer therapies, while effective in combating cancer cells, sometimes have a slew of adverse effects. Herbal treatments, with their diverse array of bioactive ingredients, can play an important role in reducing these adverse effects. Herbs such as ginger and peppermint, for example, may relieve nausea caused by chemotherapy, not only offering comfort but also improving the patient's general quality of life throughout treatment.

3. Immune Function Support

A strong immune system is essential in the body's fight against cancer. Immunomodulatory herbal therapies, such as echinacea and astragalus, can supplement conventional treatments by boosting and optimizing the immune response. This combined strategy may result in a less favorable environment for cancer development and recurrence.

4. Inflammation and Oxidative Stress Reduction

Cancer development is characterized by chronic inflammation and oxidative damage. Conventional medicines target cancer cells directly, but natural remedies like turmeric and green tea help by treating inflammation and oxidative stress. This integrated technique offers a more thorough attack on the elements that contribute to cancer development.

5. Customizing Treatment Plans

Every person's cancer journey is unique, and a one-size-fits-all strategy may not be best. The use of herbal medicines enables a more tailored treatment plan that takes into account not just the precise kind and stage of cancer but also the individual's overall health, lifestyle, and preferences. This individualized approach recognizes the complexities of cancer and tailors therapies accordingly.

6. Promoting Patient Empowerment

Patients are empowered in their recovery journey when herbal therapies and conventional treatments work together. Actively using herbal treatments promotes a sense of agency and engagement in one's own health. Patients become active participants in their treatment, contributing to their total well-being not just medically, but also emotionally and intellectually.

7. Addressing the Whole Person

Cancer is a multifaceted experience that transcends the physical realm. Integrating herbal therapies with conventional treatments takes into account and addresses the entire person—physically, emotionally, and cognitively. This holistic approach, which recognizes the interconnection of multiple facets of well-being, resonates with the developing landscape of cancer care.

The value of mixing herbs with conventional cancer therapies is enormous. It symbolizes a transition toward an integrated healing model that recognizes the benefits of both traditional and modern techniques. As we negotiate the intricacies of cancer, this collaborative method shines as a light of hope, pointing the way to comprehensive and patient-centered treatment.

Chapter 3

Specific Herbs with Anti-Cancer Properties

While certain plants have shown promise in preclinical trials or have been used traditionally for cancer treatment, the effectiveness and safety of herbal medicines for cancer treatment varies. Before introducing herbs into your treatment plan, it is critical to talk with a healthcare practitioner. Here are a few herbs that have gotten a lot of interest in cancer research:

1. Turmeric (Curcumin):

Properties: It is well-known for its anti-inflammatory and antioxidant effects.

Research: Curcumin may limit cancer cell proliferation and improve chemotherapy efficiency, according to research.

2. Ginger:

Properties: Anti-inflammatory and anti-nausea.

Research: Ginger has been proven in laboratory experiments to have anti-cancer properties and may help reduce chemotherapy-induced nausea.

3. Green Tea:

Properties: Polyphenols, notably catechins having antioxidant qualities, are abundant.

Research: Green tea has been studied for its potential in cancer therapy and has been shown in certain trials to have cancer-preventive properties.

4. Essiac Tea:

Components: A herbal combination that includes burdock root, sheep sorrel, slippery elm, and Indian rhubarb root.

Traditional Use: Essiac tea has been used in traditional medicine and has acquired favor as a cancer alternative treatment.

5. Graviola (Soursop):

Properties: High in bioactive chemicals and antioxidants.

Research: Although laboratory studies indicate possible anti-cancer properties, additional study is required.

6. Maitake and Shiitake Mushrooms:

Properties: Polysaccharides high in beta-glucans are thought to have immune-boosting properties.

Research: Some research suggests that it may have anti-cancer and immune-boosting qualities.

7. Ashwagandha:

Properties: Anti-inflammatory adaptogenic herb.

Research: According to research, ashwagandha may have anti-cancer properties and might help reduce stress.

8. Cat's Claw (Uncaria tomentosa):

Properties: Anti-inflammatory and antioxidant properties.

Research: Although laboratory studies indicate possible anti-cancer capabilities, additional clinical study is required.

9. Artemisinin (Sweet Wormwood):

Properties: Derived from the anti-malarial plant Artemisia annua.

Research: Studies have been conducted to investigate its potential anti-cancer properties, particularly when combined with conventional therapy.

10. Milk Thistle:

Properties: This product contains silymarin, which is recognized for its antioxidant and anti-inflammatory qualities.

Research: Some studies show that some cancer treatments may have a protective impact on the liver.

11. Cannabidiol (CBD):

Properties: Cannabis-derived non-psychoactive chemical.

Research: According to certain research, CBD may have anti-cancer properties and may improve the efficiency of chemotherapy.

12. Astragalus:

Properties: Known for its anti-inflammatory and immune-boosting qualities.

Research: Laboratory studies indicate possible anti-cancer properties, notably in immune system support.

Important Considerations:

Consultation: Before introducing herbs into your treatment plan, always speak with a healthcare practitioner.

Individual Variability: Individual responses to herbs might vary, and what works for one person may not work for another.

Potential Interactions: Some plants may react negatively with drugs or therapies, stressing the significance of seeking expert advice.

Integrative Approach: Herbal medicines should be used in addition to, not in instead of, conventional therapies. Herbalists and healthcare professionals work together to create an integrated approach.

Herbal medicine is a dynamic area, and current research continues to investigate the possible advantages and hazards of many herbs in cancer therapy. Always emphasize evidence-based procedures and seek individualized advice from your healthcare team.

Chapter 4

10 Herbal Infusions and Decoctions for Cancer Treatment

Below are 10 herbal infusions and decoctions, each with a step-by-step guide, measurements, dosage, and frequency. Please note that individual responses to herbs can vary, and it's important for individuals to consult with healthcare professionals before incorporating these remedies, especially if they are undergoing cancer treatment.

1. Turmeric Infusion:

Ingredients:

- 1 teaspoon of ground turmeric

- 1 cup of hot water

Steps:

1. Boil one cup of water.

2. Add 1 teaspoon of ground turmeric to the hot water.

3. Steep for 10 minutes.

4. Strain and enjoy.

Dosage and Frequency:

- Dosage: 1-2 cups per day.

- Frequency: Daily.

2. Ginger Lemon Decoction:

Ingredients:

- 1 tablespoon of fresh grated ginger

- 1 tablespoon of fresh lemon juice

- 1 cup of hot water

Steps:

1. Boil one cup of water.

2. Add grated ginger to the hot water.

3. Simmer for 10 minutes.

4. Strain and add fresh lemon juice.

5. Enjoy warm.

Dosage and Frequency:

- Dosage: 1-2 cups per day.

- Frequency: Daily.

3. Chamomile Lavender Infusion:

Ingredients:

- 1 tablespoon of dried chamomile flowers

- 1 teaspoon of dried lavender flowers

- 1 cup of hot water

Steps:

1. Boil one cup of water.

2. Place chamomile and lavender flowers in a teapot.

3. Pour hot water over the herbs.

4. Steep for 5-7 minutes.

5. Strain and enjoy.

Dosage and Frequency:

- Dosage: 1 cup before bedtime.

- Frequency: Daily.

4. Green Tea Echinacea Infusion:

Ingredients:

- 1 green tea bag

- 1 teaspoon of dried echinacea root

- 1 cup of hot water

Steps:

1. Steep the green tea bag and dried echinacea root in hot water.

2. Steep for 5-7 minutes.

3. Remove the tea bag and strain.

4. Enjoy warm.

Dosage and Frequency:

- Dosage: 1-2 cups per day.

- Frequency: Daily.

5. Peppermint Licorice Root Decoction:

Ingredients:

- 1 tablespoon of dried peppermint leaves

- 1 teaspoon of dried licorice root

- 1 cup of hot water

Steps:

1. Boil one cup of water.

2. Add peppermint leaves and licorice root to the hot water.

3. Simmer for 10 minutes.

4. Strain and enjoy.

Dosage and Frequency:

- Dosage: 1 cup after meals.

- Frequency: Daily.

6. Rosehip Hibiscus Infusion:

Ingredients:

- 1 tablespoon of dried rosehip

- 1 tablespoon of dried hibiscus flowers

- 1 cup of hot water

Steps:

1. Boil one cup of water.

2. Add dried rosehip and hibiscus flowers to the hot water.

3. Steep for 10 minutes.

4. Strain and enjoy.

Dosage and Frequency:

- Dosage: 1-2 cups per day.

- Frequency: Daily.

7. Nettle Leaf Parsley Decoction:

Ingredients:

- 1 tablespoon of dried nettle leaves

- 1 tablespoon of fresh parsley

- 1 cup of hot water

Steps:

1. Boil one cup of water.

2. Add dried nettle leaves and fresh parsley to the hot water.

3. Simmer for 10 minutes.

4. Strain and enjoy.

Dosage and Frequency:

- Dosage: 1 cup in the morning.

- Frequency: Daily.

8. Lemon Balm Valerian Root Infusion:

Ingredients:

- 1 tablespoon of dried lemon balm leaves

- 1 teaspoon of dried valerian root

- 1 cup of hot water

Steps:

1. Boil one cup of water.

2. Add dried lemon balm leaves and valerian root to the hot water.

3. Steep for 10 minutes.

4. Strain and enjoy.

Dosage and Frequency:

- Dosage: 1 cup before bedtime.

- Frequency: Daily.

9. Dandelion Root Burdock Decoction:

Ingredients:

- 1 tablespoon of dried dandelion root

- 1 tablespoon of dried burdock root

- 1 cup of hot water

Steps:

1. Boil one cup of water.

2. Add dried dandelion root and burdock root to the hot water.

3. Simmer for 15 minutes.

4. Strain and enjoy.

Dosage and Frequency:

- Dosage: 1 cup in the afternoon.

- Frequency: Daily.

10. Fennel Seed Fenugreek Infusion:

Ingredients:

- 1 tablespoon of fennel seeds

- 1 teaspoon of fenugreek seeds

- 1 cup of hot water

Steps:

1. Boil one cup of water.

2. Add fennel seeds and fenugreek seeds to the hot water.

3. Steep for 10 minutes.

4. Strain and enjoy.

Dosage and Frequency:

- Dosage: 1 cup after meals.

- Frequency: Daily.

Remember to monitor individual reactions and consult with healthcare professionals for personalized guidance. Additionally, individuals undergoing cancer treatment should inform their healthcare team about any herbal remedies they plan to incorporate into their regimen.

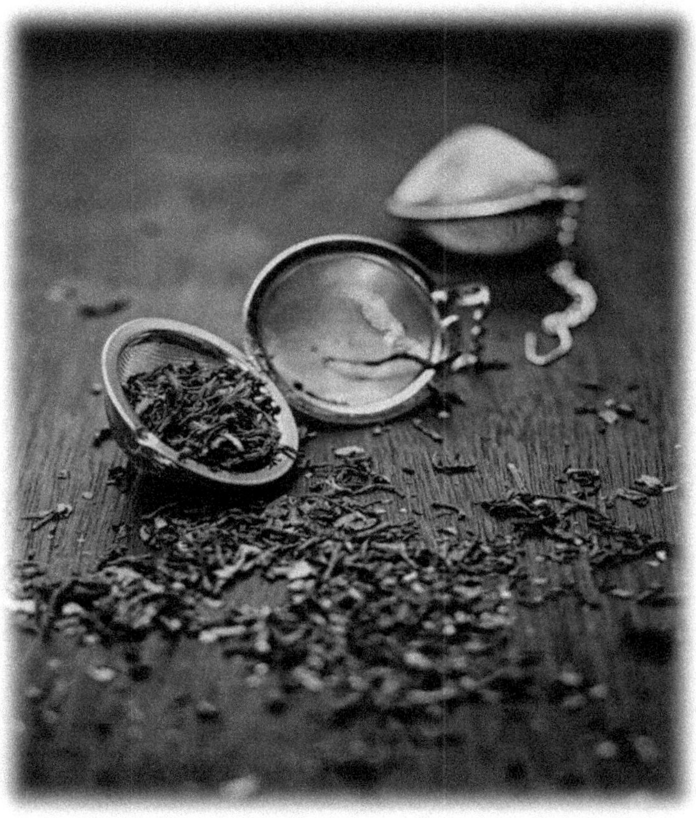

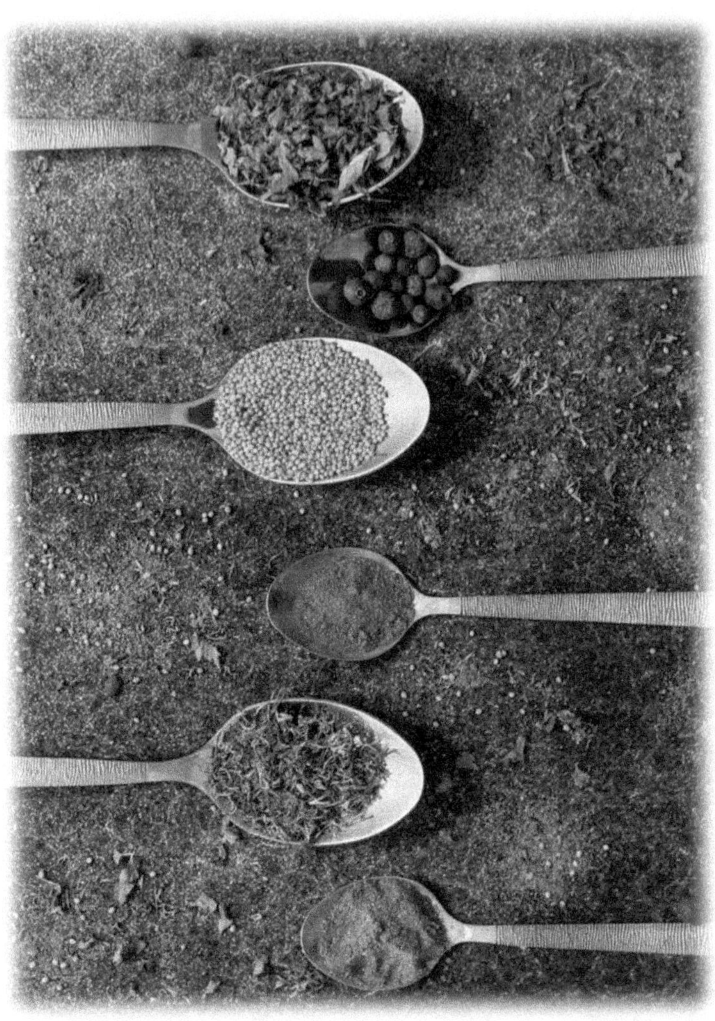

Chapter 5

Principles of an Anti-Cancer Diet

Adopting an anti-cancer diet entails combining concepts that emphasize feeding the body, strengthening the immune system, and decreasing risk factors. While nutrition cannot guarantee cancer prevention or treatment, it does play an important part in overall health promotion and may lead to a decreased risk of specific cancers. Here are some guidelines for developing an anti-cancer diet:

1. Plant-Based Emphasis:

Include a Colorful Variety of Vegetables and Fruits: Aim for a colorful variety of veggies and fruits to guarantee a wide range of nutrients and antioxidants.

Cruciferous Vegetables: Include cancer-fighting vegetables such as broccoli, cauliflower, Brussels sprouts, kale, and cabbage.

2. Whole Grains and Legumes:

Select Whole Grains: Choose whole grains over refined grains such as brown rice, quinoa, and oats. These are high in fiber and important nutrients.

Include Legumes: Plant-based protein and fiber are abundant in beans, lentils, and peas.

3. Healthy Fats

Embrace Omega-3 Fatty Acids: Include omega-3 sources such as flaxseeds, chia seeds, walnuts, and fatty fish in your diet. These lipids are anti-inflammatory in nature.

Select Olive Oil: Extra virgin olive oil is a good source of monounsaturated fats.

4. Lean Proteins:

Prioritize Lean Sources: Choose lean protein sources such as poultry, fish, tofu, lentils, and nuts as your first choice.

Reduce your intake of red and processed meats: Reduce your intake of red and processed meats, which have been linked to an elevated risk of some malignancies.

5. Limit Processed and Sugary meals:

Reduce Added Sugars: Limit your consumption of sugary beverages, sweets, and processed meals that are rich in added sugars.

Reduce Processed Foods: Reduce your consumption of processed and packaged foods, which may include preservatives and additives.

6. Hydration:

Water should be prioritized: Stay hydrated by drinking lots of water throughout the day. Limit your intake of sugary drinks and excessive caffeine.

7. Moderate Alcohol Consumption

Limit your alcohol consumption: Limit your alcohol consumption. Alcoholism has been related to an increased risk of some malignancies.

8. Herbs and Spices:

Utilize Turmeric: Turmeric contains curcumin, which has anti-inflammatory effects. Consider using turmeric in cooking or as a supplement.

Add Garlic and Ginger : These offer anti-cancer qualities and can improve the flavor of your food.

9. Foods High in Antioxidants:

Berries and Citrus Fruits: Berries are high in antioxidants, while citrus fruits are high in vitamin C, which helps the immune system.

Green Tea: Green tea, known for its polyphenols, has antioxidant effects.

10. Portion Control and careful Eating:

Practice Portion Control: To maintain a healthy weight, be careful of portion sizes.

Eat Mindfully: Pay attention to hunger and fullness cues, and relish your meals' flavors and sensations.

11 Achieve and Maintain a Healthy Weight:

Achieve and Maintain a Healthy Weight: Obesity raises the risk of various malignancies. To obtain a healthy weight, strike a balance between nutrition and physical exercise.

12 Remain Informed and Adapt:

Stay Current on Nutritional Research: Keep up with nutrition and cancer prevention research. Adapt your diet depending on new research.

13. Individualization:

Consider Individual Requirements: Recognize that everyone's nutritional demands are different. Age, gender, pre-existing health issues, and personal preferences should all be considered.

14. Consult with Healthcare Professionals:

Seek Professional Guidance: If you are receiving cancer treatment, consult with healthcare specialists, including a qualified dietitian, to develop a tailored anti-cancer food plan.

Adopting these principles as part of a holistic lifestyle that includes regular exercise, stress management, and the avoidance of tobacco products might help to improve general health and well-being, perhaps lowering the risk of some malignancies. Always seek specialized advice from healthcare specialists, especially if you have specific health problems or are receiving medical treatment.

Healthy Food You Should be Eating

A nutritious and well-balanced diet is essential for general health and well-being. A varied diet rich in nutrients supplies necessary vitamins, minerals, antioxidants, and other nutrients that support diverse biological activities. Here is a list of foods that are usually thought to be healthy:

1. Fruits:

Berries: Antioxidants are abundant in blueberries, strawberries, and raspberries.

Citrus Fruits: Citrus fruits such as oranges, lemons, and grapefruits are high in vitamin C.

Bananas:High in potassium and energy.

Apples: Rich in fiber and antioxidants.

2. Vegetables:

Leafy Greens: Spinach, kale, and Swiss chard are high in vitamins and minerals.

 Cruciferous Vegetables: Broccoli, cauliflower, and Brussels sprouts have anti-cancer chemicals.

Carrots: High in beta-carotene, which is beneficial to eye health.

Sweet Potatoes: High in fiber and vitamins.

3. Whole Grains:

Quinoa: A complete protein and fiber-rich grain.

Brown Rice: High in fiber and vitamins.

Oats: Beta-glucans are advantageous to heart health.

Whole Wheat: A good source of fiber and B vitamins.

4. Lean Proteins:

Chicken Breast: High-quality protein with a low fat content.

Fish: Omega-3 fatty acids are abundant in fatty fish such as salmon and mackerel.

Legumes and Beans: Lentils, chickpeas, and black beans are high in protein and fiber.

Tofu: A protein source derived from plants.

5. Dairy Alternatives:

Greek Yogurt: High in protein and probiotics.

Milk (or Fortified Plant-Based Milks): Calcium and vitamin D rich.

Cheese: Moderate consumption for calcium and protein.

6. Healthy Fats:

Avocado: A source of monounsaturated fats and other nutrients.

Olive Oil: High in monounsaturated fats, which are good for your heart.

Nuts and Seeds: Almonds, walnuts, and chia seeds are high in healthful fats.

7. Herbs and Spices:

Turmeric: This spice contains curcumin, which has anti-inflammatory qualities.

Cinnamon: May aid with blood sugar regulation.

Garlic: Has a variety of health advantages, including the possibility of cardiovascular benefits.

Ginger: This spice is well-known for its anti-nausea and anti-inflammatory qualities.

8. Beverages:

Water: Water is necessary for hydration and general wellness.

Green Tea: High in antioxidants and linked to a variety of health benefits.

Herbal Teas: Peppermint and chamomile for digestion and relaxation.

Coffee: In moderation, coffee may have antioxidant properties.

9. Colorful Vegetables:

Bell Peppers: Vitamin C-rich.

Tomatoes: High in lycopene, which has been linked to cancer-fighting effects.

Eggplant: Fiber and antioxidants are included in this vegetable.

10 Probiotic-Rich Foods:

Yogurt with Live Cultures: Aids in intestinal health.

Sauerkraut: Fermented foods aid in the maintenance of a healthy gut microbiota.

Kefir: A probiotic-rich fermented milk drink.

11 Dark Chocolate:

Moderate Consumption It contains antioxidants and may improve your mood.

12. Eggs:

High in Protein: Provide vital amino acids as well as other nutrients.

13. Sea Vegetables:

Seaweed: Contains iodine and other nutrients.

14. Berries:

Antioxidant-rich: Blueberries, strawberries, and raspberries.

15. Legumes:

Lentils, chickpeas, and black beans are high in fiber and protein.

Individual nutritional needs vary, therefore it's best to get tailored nutrition advice from a healthcare expert or a licensed dietitian. Moderation, portion management, and including a variety of foods into your diet all contribute to a well-rounded and healthful eating habit.

Foods You should Avoid

Some foods may lead to health problems when taken in excess or as part of an unbalanced diet. It's crucial to remember that everyone's reactions to food differ, and what's "bad" for one person may not be the same for another. Furthermore, moderation is essential, and the occasional indulgence in less healthful meals is often allowed. Here are several foods that, when taken in excess, may have detrimental health consequences:

1. Processed Foods:

Fast Food: High in harmful fats, salt, and frequently lacking in nutrients.

Packaged Snacks: Many of these snacks have extra sweets, harmful fats, and preservatives.

Processed Meats: Bacon, sausages, and deli meats are frequently rich in salt and include preservatives.

2. Sugary Foods and Beverages:

Soda and Sugary Drinks: High in added sugars, which can lead to weight gain and other health problems.

Candy and Sweets: Excess sugar consumption has been related to a variety of health issues, including tooth decay and obesity.

Pastries and Desserts: These foods frequently include excessive levels of processed sugars and harmful fats.

3. Trans Fats:

Fried Foods: Deep-fried foods may include trans fats, which elevate bad cholesterol while decreasing good cholesterol.

Baked Goods for Sale: Trans fats may be included in some cakes, cookies, and crackers.

4. Highly Refined Carbohydrates:

White Bread: Does not include the fiber and minerals present in whole grains.

White Rice: Does not include the fiber and nutrients found in brown or whole grain rice.

Pastries and Baked Goods: These are frequently produced using refined flour.

5. Highly Salted Foods:

Processed Foods: Many processed foods are rich in salt, including canned soups and snacks.

Fast Food: Excessive salt content is common.

6. Highly Processed Vegetable Oils:

Soybean Oil, Corn Oil:** High in omega-6 fatty acids, which can lead to inflammation if there is an imbalance.

Margarine: Contains trans fats often.

7. Alcohol:

Excessive Consumption: Can lead to a variety of health problems, including liver damage and an increased risk of some malignancies.

High-Calorie Cocktails: Cocktail mixers and additional sweeteners can contribute to weight gain.

8. Artificial Sweeteners:

Diet Sodas: According to certain research, artificial sweeteners may have detrimental health impacts.

No-Sugar Snacks: Artificial sweeteners may be present and should be eaten in moderation.

9. Excessive Red and Processed Meats:

Bacon, Sausages, and Hot Dogs: Preservatives associated to health risks may be found in processed meats.

Fatty Red Meat Cuts: Excessive intake may be linked to a variety of health problems.

10. Excessive Consumption of Caffeine and Energy Drinks: This can result in an elevated heart rate, sleeplessness, and other health problems.

11. Excessive Full-Fat Dairy:

Whole Milk and Full-Fat Cheese: High in saturated fats, which, when ingested in excess, may lead to cardiovascular problems.

12. Highly Sweetened Breakfast Cereals:

High in Sugar: Some cereals targeted to youngsters may contain a lot of sugar.

13. Extremely Salty Snacks:

Potato Chips and Pretzels: High in salt and, if taken in excess, may contribute to hypertension.

14. Excessive Consumption of High-Calorie Foods:

Overeating: Consuming more calories than the body requires might result in weight gain and other health problems.

15. Added Preservatives in Canned Foods:

Salt Content: Canned soups, vegetables, and other foods may have significant levels of added salt.

It is essential to approach nutrition with caution and to take into account individual health problems and dietary requirements. A well-balanced diet rich in nutrient-dense foods, along with frequent physical exercise, is essential for overall health and preventing nutritional deficiencies. If you have special dietary problems or conditions, you should get tailored advice from a healthcare expert or a qualified dietitian.

Chapter 6

10 Flavourful Breakfast Recipes that Fights Cancer

Creating nutritious and flavorful breakfast options that incorporate herbs and cancer-fighting ingredients can be a delightful way to start the day. Here are 10 breakfast ideas along with their ingredients, measurements, and preparation methods:

1. Turmeric and Berry Smoothie Bowl:

Ingredients:

- 1 cup of mixed berries such as blueberries, strawberries, raspberries

- 1 frozen banana

- 1/2 teaspoon ground turmeric

- 1 tablespoon chia seeds

- 1 cup almond milk (or any preferred milk)

Preparation:

1. Blend mixed berries, frozen banana, ground turmeric, chia seeds, and almond milk until smooth.

2. Pour into a bowl and top with additional berries, nuts, and seeds.

2. Oatmeal with Ginger and Apple Compote:

Ingredients:

- 1/2 cup rolled oats

- 1 cup milk of choice or water

- 1/2 teaspoon grated ginger

- 1 apple, diced

- 1 tablespoon honey or maple syrup

Preparation:

1. Cook rolled oats with water or milk until creamy.

2. In a separate pan, sauté grated ginger and diced apple until soft.

3. Mix the ginger-apple compote into the oatmeal and sweeten with honey or maple syrup.

3. Avocado Toast with Turmeric and Radishes:

Ingredients:

- 1 slice whole-grain bread

- 1/2 ripe avocado

- 1/2 teaspoon ground turmeric

- Sliced radishes

- Salt and pepper to taste

Preparation:

1. Toast the whole-grain bread slice.

2. Mash the ripe avocado and spread it over the toast.

3. Sprinkle ground turmeric, top with sliced radishes, and season with salt and pepper.

4. Greek Yogurt Parfait with Berries and Almonds:

Ingredients:

- 1/2 cup Greek yogurt

- 1/4 cup granola

- Mixed berries (strawberries, blueberries)

- 1 tablespoon sliced almonds

Preparation:

1. In a glass or bowl, layer Greek yogurt, granola, and mixed berries.

2. Repeat the layers and top with sliced almonds.

5. Herbal Infused Quinoa Porridge:

Ingredients:

- 1/2 cup quinoa, rinsed

- 1 cup milk of choice or water

- 1 teaspoon of dried lavender (or chamomile) flowers

- 1 tablespoon honey or maple syrup

Preparation:

1. Cook quinoa with water or milk until fluffy.

2. In the last few minutes of cooking, add dried lavender (or chamomile) flowers.

3. Sweeten with honey or maple syrup.

6. Chia Seed Pudding with Mango and Mint:

Ingredients:

- 2 tablespoons chia seeds

- 1/2 cup almond milk

- 1/2 teaspoon fresh mint, chopped

- 1/2 cup diced mango

Preparation:

1. Mix chia seeds with almond milk and let it sit in the refrigerator for at least 2 hours or overnight.

2. Before serving, stir in fresh mint and top with diced mango.

7. Egg and Spinach Breakfast Wrap with Turmeric Sauce:

Ingredients:

- 1 whole-grain wrap

- 2 eggs, scrambled

- Handful of fresh spinach

- 1/2 teaspoon ground turmeric

- Yogurt or tahini sauce

Preparation:

1. Scramble eggs and sauté fresh spinach until wilted.

2. Fill the whole-grain wrap with the eggs, spinach, and drizzle with turmeric sauce.

8. Fruit Salad with Mint and Honey-Lime Dressing:

Ingredients:

- Assorted seasonal fruits (e.g., melon, berries, kiwi)

- Fresh mint leaves, chopped

- Juice of 1 lime

- 1 tablespoon honey

Preparation:

1. Dice the assorted fruits and mix in a bowl.

2. In a small bowl, whisk together lime juice and honey.

3. Pour the dressing over the fruit salad and sprinkle with fresh mint.

9. Buckwheat Pancakes with Blueberry Compote:

Ingredients:

- 1/2 cup buckwheat flour

- 1/2 teaspoon baking powder

- 1/2 cup almond milk

- Blueberry compote (blueberries, lemon juice, honey)

Preparation:

1. In a bowl, mix buckwheat flour, baking powder, and almond milk until smooth.

2. Cook small pancakes on a griddle.

3. Serve with a blueberry compote made by simmering blueberries with lemon juice and honey.

10. Cancer-Fighting Smoothie:

Ingredients:

- 1 cup kale or spinach

- 1/2 cucumber, peeled and sliced

- 1/2 cup pineapple chunks

- 1/2 inch fresh ginger, peeled

- 1 cup coconut water

Preparation:

1. Blend kale (or spinach), cucumber, pineapple, fresh ginger, and coconut water until smooth.

2. Pour into a glass and enjoy this nutrient-packed smoothie.

Remember to customize these recipes based on individual preferences and dietary restrictions. Additionally, consulting with healthcare professionals can provide personalized guidance, especially for those undergoing cancer treatment.

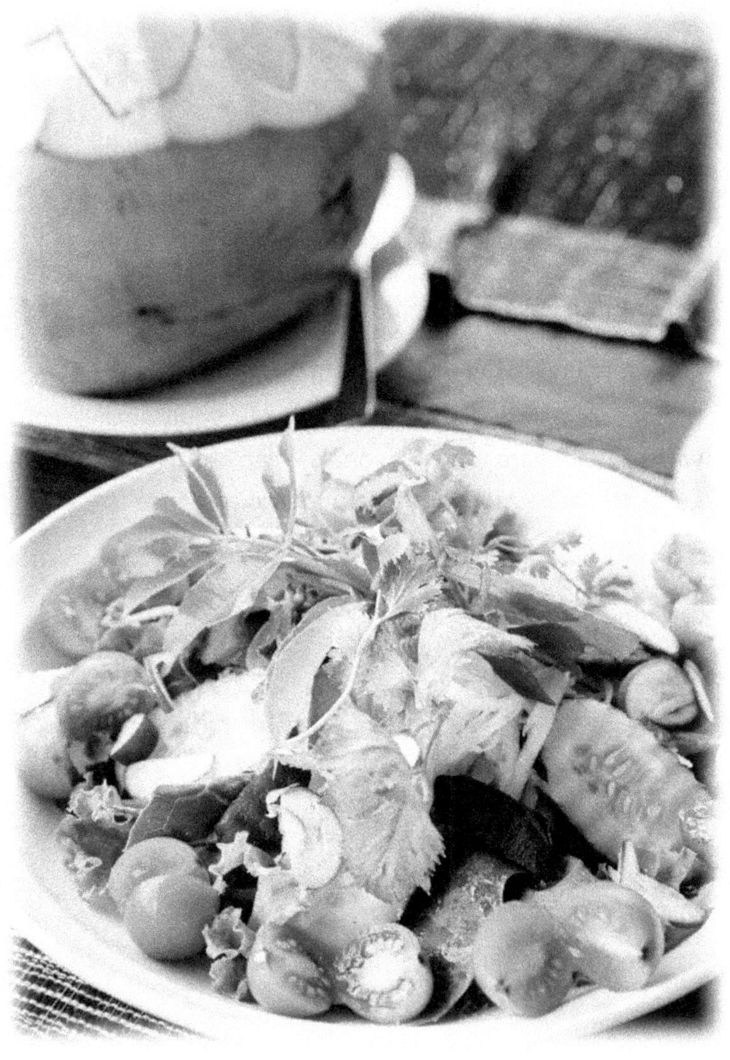

Chapter 7

10 Flavourful Lunch Recipes that Fights Cancer

Crafting nutritious and flavorful lunch recipes that incorporate cancer-fighting ingredients and herbs can contribute to a well-rounded and satisfying meal. Here are 10 unique lunch ideas, complete with ingredients, measurements, and preparation methods:

1. Salmon and Quinoa Stuffed Bell Peppers:

Ingredients:

- 2 bell peppers, divide into halve and remove seeds

- 1 cup cooked quinoa

- 6 oz cooked and flaked salmon fillet

- 1 cup cherry tomatoes, halved

- 1/4 cup feta cheese, crumbled

- Fresh dill, chopped

Preparation:

1. Preheat the oven to 375°F (190°C).

2. In a bowl, mix cooked quinoa, flaked salmon, cherry tomatoes, feta cheese, and chopped fresh dill.

3. Stuff the bell peppers with the mixture and bake for 20-25 minutes or until peppers are tender.

2. Turmeric Lentil Soup:

Ingredients:

- 1 cup red lentils, rinsed

- 1 onion, chopped

- 2 carrots, diced

- 2 teaspoons ground turmeric

- 4 cups vegetable broth

- Fresh cilantro, chopped

Preparation:

1. In a pot, sauté onions and carrots until softened.

2. Add red lentils, ground turmeric, and vegetable broth. Bring to a boil.

3. Simmer until lentils are cooked, and flavors meld. Garnish with chopped cilantro.

3. Chickpea and Spinach Salad with Lemon-Tahini Dressing:

Ingredients:

- 1 can chickpeas, drained and rinsed

- 2 cups fresh spinach

- 1 cucumber, diced

- 1/4 cup red onion, finely chopped

- Dressing: 2 tablespoons tahini, juice of 1 lemon, salt, and pepper

Preparation:

1. Combine chickpeas, fresh spinach, diced cucumber, and chopped red onion in a bowl.

2. Whisk together tahini, lemon juice, salt, and pepper for the dressing.

3. Toss the salad with the dressing before serving.

4. Mushroom and Turmeric Brown Rice Risotto:

Ingredients:

- 1 cup brown rice

- 2 cups mushrooms, sliced

- 1 onion, finely chopped

- 1 teaspoon ground turmeric

- 4 cups vegetable broth

- Parmesan cheese (optional)

Preparation:

1. In a pan, sauté onions until translucent, add mushrooms and cook until browned.

2. Add brown rice, ground turmeric, and vegetable broth. Simmer until rice is cooked.

3. Garnish with Parmesan cheese if desired.

5. Grilled Chicken and Quinoa Salad with Herb Vinaigrette:

Ingredients:

- 1 cup cooked quinoa

- Grilled chicken breast, sliced

- Mixed salad greens

- Cherry tomatoes, halved

- Herbs (parsley, basil, chives), chopped

- Vinaigrette: Olive oil, balsamic vinegar, Dijon mustard, salt, and pepper

Preparation:

1. Combine cooked quinoa, grilled chicken, mixed greens, cherry tomatoes, and chopped herbs in a bowl.

2. Whisk together olive oil, balsamic vinegar, Dijon mustard, salt, and pepper for the vinaigrette.

3. Drizzle the salad with the vinaigrette before serving.

6. Cauliflower and Turmeric Soup:

Ingredients:

- 1 cauliflower, chopped

- 1 onion, diced

- 2 teaspoons ground turmeric

- 4 cups vegetable broth

- Coconut milk (optional)

- Fresh coriander, chopped

Preparation:

1. In a pot, sauté onions until softened, add chopped cauliflower and ground turmeric.

2. Pour in vegetable broth and simmer until cauliflower is tender.

3. Blend the soup until smooth, add coconut milk if desired, and garnish with fresh coriander.

7. Sweet Potato and Ginger Stir-Fry:

Ingredients:

- 2 sweet potatoes, peeled and cubed

- 1 bell pepper, sliced

- 1 cup broccoli florets

- 2 tablespoons fresh ginger, grated

- 1 tablespoon soy sauce

- Brown rice (optional)

Preparation:

1. Steam or boil sweet potatoes until slightly tender.

2. In a pan, stir-fry sweet potatoes, bell pepper, broccoli, and grated ginger until cooked.

3. Drizzle with soy sauce and serve over brown rice if desired.

8. Spinach and Walnut Pesto Pasta:

Ingredients:

- Whole wheat pasta

- 2 cups fresh spinach

- 1/2 cup walnuts

- 2 cloves garlic

- 1/4 cup grated Parmesan cheese

- Olive oil

Preparation:

1. Cook whole wheat pasta according to package instructions.

2. In a food processor, blend spinach, walnuts, garlic, Parmesan cheese, and enough olive oil to form a pesto.

3. Toss the cooked pasta with the spinach and walnut pesto.

9. Baked Herb-Crusted Salmon with Quinoa Salad:

Ingredients:

- Salmon fillets

- Herbs (dill, parsley, thyme), chopped

- Lemon zest

- Quinoa salad (quinoa, cherry tomatoes, cucumber, feta cheese)

Preparation:

1. Preheat the oven to 375°F (190°C).

2. Mix chopped herbs and lemon zest. Press onto salmon fillets.

3. Bake until salmon is cooked through. Serve with a side of quinoa salad.

10. Vegetarian Cauliflower and Chickpea Curry:

Ingredients:

- 1 cauliflower, cut into florets

- 1 can chickpeas, drained

- 1 onion, finely chopped

- 2 tomatoes, diced

- Curry spices (turmeric, cumin, coriander, chili powder)

- Coconut milk

Preparation:

1. In a pan, sauté onions until translucent. After adding the curry spices, simmer for one minute.

2. Add cauliflower, chickpeas, and diced tomatoes. Pour in coconut milk.

3. Simmer until cauliflower is tender. Serve over brown rice.

These lunch recipes are designed to be flavorful, nutritious, and incorporate cancer-fighting ingredients. Adjustments can be made based on individual preferences and dietary needs. Always consult with healthcare professionals for personalized advice, especially for those undergoing cancer treatment.

Chapter 8

10 Flavourful Dinner Recipes that Fights Cancer

Dinner is an essential part of the day, and incorporating cancer-fighting ingredients can make it both delicious and nutritious. Here are 10 dinner recipes, complete with ingredients, measurements, and preparation methods:

1. Baked Herb-Crusted Chicken with Quinoa and Roasted Vegetables:

Ingredients:

- Chicken breasts

- Herbs (rosemary, thyme, oregano), chopped

- Garlic, minced

- Olive oil

- Quinoa

- Mixed vegetables (zucchini, bell peppers, cherry tomatoes)

Preparation:

1. Preheat the oven to 400°F (200°C).

2. Mix chopped herbs, minced garlic, and olive oil. Coat chicken breasts with the mixture.

3. Bake until chicken is cooked through. Serve over cooked quinoa with roasted vegetables.

2. Cancer-Fighting Stir-Fried Tofu and Broccoli:

Ingredients:

- Firm tofu, cubed

- Broccoli florets

- Sesame oil

- Garlic, minced

- Soy sauce

- Brown rice

Preparation:

1. Press tofu to remove excess water, then stir-fry with broccoli in sesame oil.

2. Add minced garlic and soy sauce, cooking until tofu is golden brown.

3. Serve over brown rice.

3. Turmeric and Garlic Shrimp Skewers with Quinoa Salad:

Ingredients:

- Shrimp, peeled and deveined

- Turmeric

- Garlic, minced

- Lemon juice

- Quinoa salad (quinoa, cucumber, cherry tomatoes, feta cheese)

Preparation:

1. Marinate shrimp in turmeric, minced garlic, and lemon juice.

2. Thread shrimp onto skewers and grill until cooked.

3. Serve with a side of quinoa salad.

4. Mushroom and Spinach Stuffed Bell Peppers:

Ingredients:

- Bell peppers, halved and seeds removed

- Mushrooms, chopped

- Fresh spinach

- Onion, diced

- Brown rice

- Tomato sauce

Preparation:

1. Sauté mushrooms, spinach, and diced onion.

2. Mix with cooked brown rice and stuff bell peppers.

3. Bake until peppers are tender. Serve with tomato sauce.

5. Salmon and Asparagus Foil Packets with Herbs:

Ingredients:

- Salmon fillets

- Asparagus spears

- Lemon slices

- Herbs (dill, parsley), chopped

- Olive oil

Preparation:

1. Preheat the oven to 400°F (200°C).

2. Place salmon fillets and asparagus on foil sheets.

3. Drizzle with olive oil, sprinkle with chopped herbs, and add lemon slices.

4. Seal the foil packets and bake until salmon is cooked.

6. Brown Rice with Chickpea and Vegetable Curry:

Ingredients:

- 1 can chickpeas, drained

- Mixed vegetables (carrots, peas, bell peppers)

- Onion, finely chopped

- Curry spices (cumin, coriander, turmeric)

- Coconut milk

- Brown rice

Preparation:

1. Sauté onions and mixed vegetables until softened.

2. Add chickpeas, curry spices, and coconut milk. Simmer until vegetables are tender.

3. Serve over brown rice.

7. Herb-Roasted Turkey Breast with Quinoa Pilaf:

Ingredients:

- Turkey breast

- Herbs (sage, rosemary, thyme), chopped

- Garlic, minced

- Quinoa pilaf (quinoa, diced carrots, green peas)

Preparation:

1. Preheat the oven to 350°F (175°C).

2. Rub turkey breast with chopped herbs and minced garlic.

3. Roast until turkey is cooked. Serve with quinoa pilaf.

8. Vegetarian Lentil and Spinach Soup:

Ingredients:

- 1 cup lentils, rinsed

- Fresh spinach

- Carrots, diced

- Onion, finely chopped

- Vegetable broth

- Turmeric

Preparation:

1. Sauté onions and carrots until softened.

2. Add lentils, turmeric, and vegetable broth. Simmer until lentils are cooked.

3. Stir in fresh spinach just before serving.

9. Grilled Herb-Marinated Portobello Mushrooms:

Ingredients:

- Portobello mushrooms, stems removed

- Balsamic vinegar

- Olive oil

- Herbs (thyme, rosemary), chopped

- Quinoa or couscous

Preparation:

1. Whisk together balsamic vinegar, olive oil, and chopped herbs.

2. Marinate portobello mushrooms and grill until tender.

3. Serve over quinoa or couscous.

10. Eggplant and Tomato Bake with Herbed Quinoa:

Ingredients:

- Eggplant, sliced

- Cherry tomatoes, halved

- Garlic, minced

- Herbed quinoa (quinoa, parsley, basil)

Preparation:

1. Layer sliced eggplant and halved cherry tomatoes in a baking dish.

2. Sprinkle minced garlic and bake until vegetables are tender.

3. Serve over herbed quinoa.

These dinner recipes are designed to be not only flavorful but also rich in cancer-fighting ingredients. Adjustments can be made based on individual preferences and dietary needs. As always, consult with healthcare professionals for personalized advice, especially for those undergoing cancer treatment.

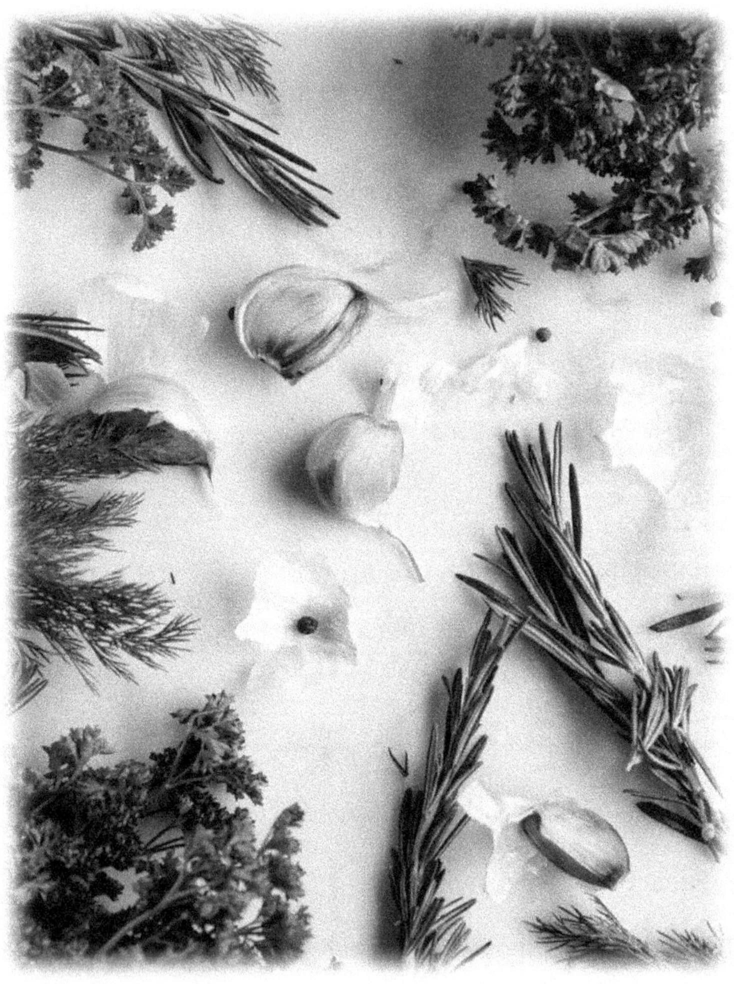

Chapter 9

Potential Side Effects of Herbal Remedies

While herbal medicines provide a variety of health advantages, it is important to be aware that they may also have negative effects, interactions, and contraindications. Here are some things to think about when it comes to the potential adverse effects of herbal remedies:

1. Allergy Reactions: Certain plants may cause allergic reactions in certain people. Allergic responses can vary from modest symptoms like skin rashes to severe ones like trouble breathing. If any indications of an allergic response appear, it is critical to quit usage.

2. Drug Interactions: Herbal medicines and prescription pharmaceuticals can interact, reducing their efficacy or increasing the risk of negative effects. To avoid potential interactions, always notify your healthcare physician about any herbal supplements you are taking.

3. Gastrointestinal Issues: Certain herbs might induce nausea, vomiting, or diarrhea. High dosages of some laxative herbs, for example, may cause gastric upset.

4. Changes in Blood Pressure: - Some herbs might affect blood pressure. Individuals with hypertension or on blood pressure drugs should exercise caution while using botanicals that may impact blood pressure levels.

5. Liver and Kidney Issues: Some herbs may have hepatotoxic or nephrotoxic effects, affecting liver or kidney function. Regular monitoring is critical, especially for people who already have liver or renal disease.

6. Pregnancy and Lactation: Pregnant or nursing women should use herbal treatments with care. Some herbs may be harmful to a growing fetus or a breastfeeding child. Before utilizing herbs during pregnancy or breastfeeding, always speak with a healthcare practitioner.

7. Photosensitivity: Some herbs might make you more sensitive to sunshine, causing skin responses. Individuals who use photosensitizing herbs should take steps to protect their skin from overexposure to the sun.

8. Bleeding Risks: Several herbs, including garlic, ginkgo biloba, and ginger, have antiplatelet or anticoagulant properties. This can raise the risk of bleeding, especially in people who use blood thinners.

9. Endocrine Disruption: Some herbs have hormonal effects and can disrupt the endocrine system. Individuals with hormonal disorders or on hormone-based drugs should exercise caution when using herbs.

10. Central Nervous System (CNS) Effects: Certain herbs may have central nervous system (CNS) effects, producing sleepiness or changing cognitive function. Individuals should use caution, particularly when driving heavy machinery or engaged in tasks that require mental awareness.

11. Additional Effects with Conventional therapies: Herbal medicines may have additive effects when taken in conjunction with conventional medical therapies. Depending on the circumstances, this might be advantageous or dangerous. It is critical to collaborate with healthcare providers.

12. Quality and Contamination Concerns: Low-quality herbal items may include pesticides, heavy metals, or other dangerous chemicals. To ensure product quality and safety, it is important to acquire herbal treatments from trustworthy providers.

13. Individual Variability: Individual reactions to herbs might differ. What works well for one individual may not work well for another. Individual responses must be monitored in order to alter dose or cease treatment if necessary.

Individuals should contact with certified healthcare specialists, such as herbalists, naturopathic physicians, or traditional healthcare practitioners, before adopting herbal therapies into a healthcare routine. Healthcare practitioners can give individualized advise based on an individual's health state, current medical issues, and probable prescription interactions. Individuals should also notify their healthcare team about any herbal supplements they are taking in order to receive thorough and coordinated care.

Common Cancer Side Effects and Natural ways to Relieve Them

Cancer and its therapies are frequently associated with a variety of side effects that can have a substantial influence on an individual's quality of life. While medical interventions are necessary, there are also natural alternatives to alleviate some of the most prevalent cancer side effects. It is crucial to emphasize that these recommendations should be evaluated with healthcare specialists to ensure that they are appropriate for particular health conditions and treatment programs.

1. Exhaustion

Natural Relief:

Gentle Exercise: To fight weariness, use gentle workouts such as walking or yoga.

Adequate Rest: Make quality sleep a priority and take short naps during the day.

Hydration: Stay hydrated to avoid weariness caused by dehydration.

2. Nausea and Vomiting:

Natural Relief:

Ginger: Drink ginger tea or take ginger supplements, which have anti-nausea effects.

Peppermint: Peppermint tea or aromatherapy may aid with nausea relief.

Miniature, Frequent Meals: To aid digestion, choose smaller, more frequent meals.

3. Pain:

Natural Relief:

Turmeric: Turmeric, known for its anti-inflammatory characteristics, may help relieve pain.

Acupuncture: Acupuncture can help with pain alleviation and overall well-being.

Heat and Cold Therapy: For alleviation, apply heat or cold packs to the afflicted regions.

4. Cognitive Impairment (Chemo Brain):

Natural Relief:

Mental Exercises: Take part in brain-stimulating activities such as puzzles or memory games.

Adequate Sleep: Maintain good sleep hygiene for optimal cognitive performance.

Mindfulness Practices: Meditation and other mindfulness practices may increase attention and mental clarity.

5. Constipation:

Natural Relief:

Fiber-Rich Foods: Eat fruits, vegetables, and whole grains.

Hydration: To soften stools, drink plenty of water.

 Workout: Regular physical exercise can aid in the stimulation of bowel motions.

6. Diarrhea:

Natural Relief:

Bananas and Rice: These might aid in stool firmness.

Probiotics: Consume probiotic-rich foods such as yogurt to improve gut health.

Hydration: To avoid dehydration, drink electrolyte-rich drinks.

7. Hair Loss:

Natural Relief:

Cold Cap Therapy: Use cold caps during chemotherapy to prevent hair loss.

Gentle Hair Care: Use gentle shampoos and avoid overheating your hair.

8. Skin Changes:

Natural Relief:

Aloe Vera Gel: Aloe vera gel soothes irritated skin.

Fragrance-Free Products: Use scent-free skincare products.

Sun Protection: Use caps and sunscreen to protect delicate skin from the sun.

9. Appetite Loss:

Natural Relief:

 Small, Nutrient-Dense Meals: Concentrate on nutrient-dense meals in smaller quantities.

Herbal Teas:

To boost hunger, drink herbal teas such as peppermint or chamomile.

Aromatherapy: Certain fragrances may aid in appetite stimulation.

10. Mood Shifts (Depression and Anxiety):

Natural Relief

Exercise: Regular physical exercise helps improve mood.

Mindfulness and Meditation: Techniques for relaxation and mindfulness.

Social Support: Talk to supportive friends and family members, or join a support group.

11. Immune System Support:

Natural Relief:

Vitamin C-Rich Foods: Citrus fruits, berries, and bell peppers are examples of vitamin C-rich foods.

Zinc: Consume foods like nuts, seeds, and legumes to boost your immune system.

Echinacea: Before utilizing this herb for immune support, consult with a healthcare provider.

It is critical to underline that these natural therapies should be used in addition to, not in instead of, medical therapy. Before implementing any new tactics into their care plan, individuals should always talk with their healthcare team. Healthcare specialists may give tailored counsel, ensuring that these treatments are safe and appropriate for each individual's situation.

Precautions and Understanding Herb-Drug Interactions

Understanding herb-specific warnings and herb-drug interactions is critical for the safe and successful use of herbal treatments. Here are some warnings for certain plants, as well as concerns for herb-drug interactions:

Echinacea (Echinacea purpurea):

Precautions:

People with autoimmune illnesses should use echinacea with caution since it may activate the immune system.

Individuals who are allergic to plants of the Asteraceae family (e.g., ragweed, marigolds) may experience allergic responses.

St. John's Wort (Hypericum perforatum):

Precautions:

St. John's Wort may interact with a variety of drugs, including antidepressants, birth control pills, and anticoagulants. Before usage, consult a healthcare practitioner.

Garlic (Allium sativum):

Precautions:

Garlic has antiplatelet properties, which may increase the risk of bleeding. Individuals on blood-thinning drugs should exercise caution.

Ginkgo Biloba (Ginkgo biloba):

Precautions:

Ginkgo biloba may raise the risk of bleeding and interact with blood-thinning drugs. Consult a healthcare professional, especially before undergoing surgery.

Ginseng (Panax ginseng, Panax quinquefolius):

Precautions:

Ginseng can have an effect on blood pressure and blood sugar levels. Ginseng should be used with caution by those who have hypertension or diabetes.

Turmeric (Curcuma longa):

Precautions:

Turmeric may have antiplatelet effects and may interact with blood thinners. Individuals on anticoagulant treatment should exercise caution.

Ginger (Zingiber officinale):

Precautions:

Ginger may have antiplatelet effects and may interact with blood thinners. Before using, consult a healthcare practitioner.

Milk Thistle (Silybum marianum):

Precautions:

Milk thistle may have hepatoprotective properties and may interfere with drugs that are metabolized by the liver. If you are taking drugs that are processed by the liver, talk to your doctor.

Valerian (Valeriana officinalis):

Precautions:

Valerian may cause drowsiness and interact with sedative drugs. When using valerian alongside sedative drugs, use caution.

Saw Palmetto (Serenoa repens):

Precautions:

Saw palmetto may interact with hormonal drugs and cause hormonal imbalances. Consult a healthcare expert, especially if you have a hormonal issue.

Hawthorn (Crataegus spp.):

Precautions:

Hawthorn may have cardiovascular effects and may interfere with cardiac medicines. Consult with a healthcare practitioner, especially if you have cardiac problems.

Herb-Drug Interactions:

Communication with Healthcare Providers:

- Inform your healthcare doctors about any herbal supplements you are using.

- Talk about potential interactions, especially if you're taking medicine for a chronic disease.

Monitoring and Adjustments:

- When mixing herbs and pharmaceuticals, regular monitoring of health factors may be required.

- Based on the combined effects of herbs and medications, healthcare practitioners may need to change prescription doses.

Documentation and research:

- Learn about herb-drug interactions from credible sources.

- Maintain a detailed record of all drugs and herbal supplements consumed.

Individuals should seek the advice of a healthcare practitioner before introducing herbal medicines into their health routine, especially if they are using prescription pharmaceuticals. Healthcare practitioners can provide individualized advice based on an individual's health state and prospective interactions. Communication with healthcare specialists on a regular basis promotes a coordinated and safe approach to health and well-being.

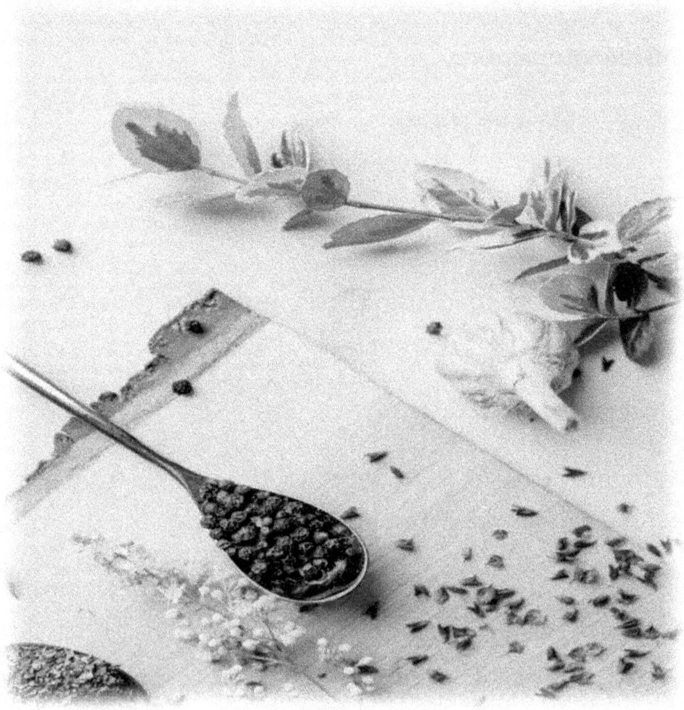

Conclusion

The resonance of hope, wisdom, and empowerment echoes through the pages as we pull the curtains on our transforming trip through A Comprehensive Guide to Herbal Remedies for Cancer. This handbook, beautifully woven with compassion and knowledge, has served as a guiding light for people traversing the difficult terrain of cancer.

At the end of this guide, we consider the power of adopting a holistic healing paradigm—one that integrates the best of ancient wisdom with current medical advances. The path has been one of discovery, unraveling cancer's riddles, comprehending its emotional tapestry, and creating a story of perseverance and hope. Readers have begun on a journey that views healing as a symphony—an delicate interplay of mind, body, and spirit.

Herbal cancer cures have been more than a guide; they have been a path to empowerment. Knowledge has been the key to unraveling the mysteries of cancer's causes, kinds, and stages. Individuals have earned a feeling of agency by adopting this information, which is a critical tool for making informed health decisions. The book has opened the path for a more confident and educated approach to cancer care by demystifying standard therapies and giving insights into controlling side effects.

The research of herbal medicines has been central to this guide—a compelling voyage into the core of nature's healing symphony. Herbal remedies' significance in cancer therapy has been highlighted, emphasizing their therapeutic potential and the need of combining these therapies with conventional techniques. The guide has acted as a link, connecting people with nature's therapeutic touch and encouraging faith in the human body's resilience.

A one-of-a-kind culinary adventure has begun, asking readers to embrace an anti-cancer diet that feeds not just the body but also the spirit. The book has produced a vivid image of a lifestyle that supports general well-being via the delightful inclusion of cancer-fighting foods and herbs into regular meals. The kitchen has become a haven for therapeutic ingredients, resulting in a symphony of tastes and wellness.

As we traverse the complexities of precautions and herb-drug interactions, the guide has stood watch, protecting its readers' health and well-being. Individuals are better able to handle their recovery path with confidence and safety after learning about the potential negative effects of herbal therapies and the necessity of communicating with healthcare experts.

A caring story at the center of this book acknowledges the emotional consequences of a cancer diagnosis. "Herbal remedies for cancer" has been a reassuring presence that understands concerns, anxieties, and the need for emotional resilience. The guide has extended a caring hand, asking readers to nurture their emotional well-being as a vital part of their recovery path, via stories of strength and coping skills.

When readers finish the final chapter of "Herbal Remedies for Cancer," they are not saying goodbye to a book, but rather moving into a more resilient future. The book goes beyond the pages, becoming a living monument to the power of knowledge, holistic medicine, and the synergistic link between nature and science. Each reader is now armed with newfound knowledge, ready to take their own route to healing.

To summarize, "Herbal remedies for cancer" is a symphony—a composition of knowledge, compassion, and empowerment. It is a testament to the human spirit's tenacity and the immense capacity for healing that each individual possesses. As this guide's echoes remain in the hearts of its readers, may they take the beautiful melody of hope and healing into their futures, embracing a life that vibrates with energy, purpose, and the symphony of well-being beyond cancer.

Other similar books that you will also like:

1. **Weight Loss Smoothies for Women Over 50**

2. **Kidney Dialysis Diet Cookbook**

3. Smoothies For Diabetes

4. Detoxification and Cleanser Diet for Women

5. Diabetic Renal Diet Cookbook

www.ingramcontent.com/pod-product-compliance
Lightning Source LLC
Chambersburg PA
CBHW071602270726

48661CB00017B/345